Exercises You Can Do in the Office, at Your Desk to Keep You Fit

Foreword

As people, we are encouraged to work hard and travel down a road of success in order to achieve our goals and end up with good occupations. These roads lead us to many places whether it's a construction area, or a lion tamer. Sometimes these roads may lead to the office life, which is a great opportunity but it may have some physical restrictions. There may be days where things are going slow. For instance, having to deal with a frustrated client, an elongated business call, and even that usual crick in your lower back from sitting up for too long. You may be dealing with different variations of psychosomatic pains and you may not know how to cope or handle the situation. The days are getting longer and you aren't getting younger, my friend; and with that being said you must learn to commit and conquer these issues with the use of daily physical exercise!

Exercising daily doesn't necessarily have to involve a gym, two hundred pound weights, and a personal fitness trainer. You can exercise in the comfort of your office using just yourself, and still get great results. Physical exercise is known to: promote proper weight control, helps you fight against health conditions and diseases, improves your overall mood, boosts energy, promotes better sleep, and helps you throw some color on a gray day by having fun. Here we will explore the many possible exercises that you can perform right in the comfort of your workspace!

It is very important to be aware of your surroundings. In this chapter we will explore the work area and figure out ways to adapt your new routine to your office. This may involve little or no rearranging, either ways, it will get you to an active start.

There is a big difference between emotional, physical, and mental stress. This chapter will help you evaluate the origin of your issues and will help you find out what you need help with most. Every person is different so this step will help benefit those who need a unique plan specially fit for them.

Chapter Three: *Here's the Exercising Part*......................................

Finally, the exercises come in to play. This chapter will show the different exercises and what they improve whether the improvement be physical, mental, emotional, or even all three. You can handpick your own personal plan from these individual workouts made for your office workspace.

Chapter Four: *Planning Goals/ Developing Healthy Habits*.............

Some people may want a six pack, others may want a simple peace of mind. Everyone has goals so we will use this chapter to help establish those goals and keep them under maintenance. This is also a bigger commitment than it seems so this will help you plan accordingly. Exercising routines also need a good diet, good attitude, etc... All of that will be discussed in the final chapter.

Chapter One

Exploring the Office Space

As you may have noticed, it may be rather difficult to perform a full blown, intense exercise routine amongst all the office items located within your office. Any and every exercise requires a decent amount of space. This will help protect you, others around you. This may involve a bit of redecorating, and that doesn't mean that you should throw your desk out the window it just means that maybe move a few chairs, tables, and plants closer to the walls so you have a clear space in the middle. To get a quick and reliable measurement that will show you whether or not you are in a safe surrounding, hold your arms out to the side and spin in a 360 degree circle. IF you did not bump or hit anything while doing so, it is safe to say that you are officially one step closer to changing your life for the better. Just as a safety precaution, take a few steps back and forth, side to side, and spin in a 360 degree circle once more to make sure that you have a comfortable workout zone.

Once that is taken care of, it is highly recommended to get a "workout matt" of some sort. If not a workout matt, a thick blanket or towel is a great substitute that will benefit in a variety of ways. The purpose is to create a better surface for you to work out on, it will provide you with:

- A softer surface that will be more comfortable overall.

- A safety cover for your floor so you won't potentially wear out the flooring and harm the office.

- An absorbent surface that will keep all bodily fluids, that may come out during extreme physical exertion (sweat, spit, etc...), off of your floor

Now that we have established the safety regulations and precautions that need to be taken it's time to discuss what you will work out in. I think we both can agree that working out in a coat jacket and khakis may look and feel a bit silly. Instead here are a few options of clothing you can wear:

- A plain, old t-shirt is a very comfortable choice as it is light material and easy to move in.

- A sleeveless shirt gives you good range of freedom for your arm and is a good choice because exercising tends to get hot.

- A tank top is very light, easy to move in, and is comfortable material overall.

- Track pants, Sweat pants help you perspire which definitely helps to get a nice workout.

- (Suggested for Women) Yoga pants or leggings because of their malleability, and flexible motion.

- Athletic shorts are definitely a choice you can't go wrong with as you can easily move, and work in comfortably.

- A thin windbreaker is good for those who really want to work up a sweat or are just feeling a bit of a draft.

As long as you are comfortable with it, you can wear virtually anything. Just make sure the clothing isn't too tight that it obstructs breathing, just tight enough to feel snug and still let your skin breathe. The goal is to feel at your prime so don't wear anything that may obstruct that vision such as:

- Dangling jewelry is a big hazard. Jewelry can potentially harm you greatly by possibly getting caught on the floor, objects around you, or even yourself which may hurt you.

- Pins and sharp objects of any kind should be avoided at all costs. The last thing you need during jumping jacks is to jump right onto a pin.

- Loose, long earrings can get caught in your hair if you are pushing yourself hard enough. Don't let cute accessories stop you from pushing yourself.

- If your hair is long, tie it in a ponytail for the time being.

- Baggy clothing may slow you down and keep you distracted.

- Thick, heavy clothing will get you hot and risk you getting overheated and that is not safe.

Now you have your space, your matt (towel, blanket, etc…), and you have your clothes. You are now fully aware of your surroundings and are officially equipped to undergo a physical, mental, and emotional transformation.

Chapter Two
Observing your Body, Mind, and Heart

How do I observe my body?

Observation is key to any process that takes place in life. You have to understand what the problem is so you can easily find a way to create a unique solution for the issue at hand. When I say observe I don't necessarily mean to just concentrate on your body just go through your regular routine and, for instance, if you start feeling aches and sore spots, pin point where they are. Everyone's body is different and unique which means we should be extra careful and very conscious of our actions and see how our own body is. When you sit in a chair, do you sit up straight or slouch? When you're walking do you drag your feet or have an energetic bounce in your step? Figuring these things out will definitely create a more accurate and beneficial solution for you.

Your body is more than just a piece meat that people look at it. Your body is an extension of your heart and mind that lets you enjoy all the good things in life. To keep your body healthy and fit you must not only exercise regularly, you must eat well, not put too much physical strain on yourself, and get plenty of rest. Even if that means switching white bread to whole wheat and shutting your eyes at night an hour earlier, it'll make a big difference that you can feel and see.

Think of your body as a home for your soul. You wouldn't want your home to be mediocre, you would work hard to furnish and make it look good for yourself. Working hard and having a determined goal will definitely help you overcome a variety of issues whether its pains, sores, or just that lethargic afternoon feeling.

Once you've discovered your body and found areas that you believe need improvement, you have officially learned explored one of the greatest gifts given to you: your body.

How do I observe my mind?

To observe your mind is a tricky thing, yet so simple. Don't focus on what you're thing or doing, just go about your day while keeping a small mental tab of how your thought process goes. People who are stressed have a bad habit of "overthinking'. This can be overthinking solutions to simple problems or overthinking to such an extent where you start to create realistic scenarios that usually have a negative response on the body. It will basically be you harming your own body out of stress, which in turn will only be adding more stress. You can easily stop these stress issues if you distract your mind with something more beneficial, fun, and healthy: exercise!

When a day is dragging on, we tend to get cranky and not have the best thoughts. Negativity can plague the mind and cause a stain to come upon your personality. People may not want such a negative person around them, even though it's not your fault that you have to work so much and deal with all the diverse variables of the office life.

You must make sure you take note of the things you say and think about because it will help you realize what is going on in the deep, mysterious crevices of your mind.

How do I observe my heart?

The human heart is a complex organ that keeps you moving, but metaphorically, it is much more. It is an emotional bank of feelings that has different chambers and locks and mechanisms that create you as a person. This "emotional bank" can be affected by how much you withdraw from it, and we all know that taking too much can leave you empty.

To observe your heart means that you have to observe your true character as a person and really dig deep. You must think about what you want from life and who you are. What are your relationships with friends and coworkers like? Is there any trouble with some loved ones? What are your goals? Everything must be taken into account to create a more accurate representation of how you are doing in order to create a workout that will benefit you.

How does observing my body, mind, and heart help with exercising?

Exercising is more than just a series of movements used to get a great physique. Exercise is a way to escape everything. It lets you leave all the worldly objects, people, and pressure that may be daunting you. It lets you come back to your basic instincts and helps you improve yourself which can help you feel and look better. It gives you a cause that you may not have. If you're stressed, you can vent it through exercising in a healthy and fun way.

You can benefit your body by being healthier and looking great!

You can benefit your mind by having more peace since you can vent through the exercises.

You can benefit your heart by making it stronger and allowing you to focus more on yourself which helps you be better with others.

Chapter Three

Here's the Exercising Part

Finally, the moment you've been waiting for, the exercises!

Exercising is fun and beneficial, but you can maximize the level of efficiency by using what you need by setting a routine and not just doing everything all at once. Each exercise focuses on a certain aspect of the body. I will help you recognize basic exercises and how they can benefit you.

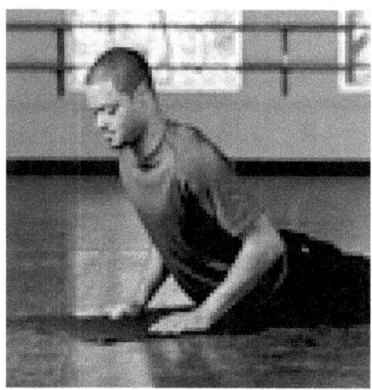

"Cobra"- This exercise is a great stretcher that targets your abs and your back. Lie on your stomach on an exercise mat or floor with your hands positioned directly under your shoulders and fingers facing forward. Legs should be straight and toes pointed. Gently exhale. Engage your abdominal/core muscles to support the spine. Press your hips into the mat or floor. Lengthen the torso and curl your chest away from the ground while keeping your hips stable. Keep the shoulders rolling down and back. Hold this position for 15 - 30 seconds. Downward Phase: Gently lower your upper body back to the mat or floor, lengthening the spine as you descend. If you experience any pain in the low back with this movement, stop the exercise immediately and consult with your doctor.

As the length of arms differ, individuals may often lift their hips off the mat or floor as they fully extend their arms. In this case, limit the extension in your arms to keep the hips on the mat.

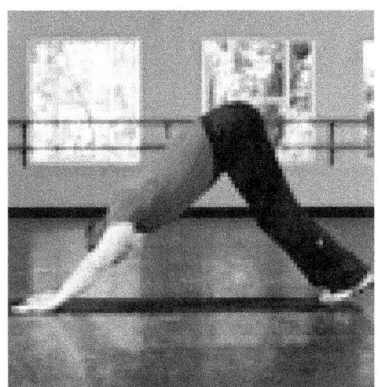

"Downward Dog Stretch"- This nice stretch focuses on your arms, back, hips, calves and shins, and thighs. Come to an all-fours position on the floor mat, with your hands under your shoulders hands fingers facing forward. Engaging your abdominals to support the spine, step back one foot at a time, coming to a push-up position (plank). Your hands should remain under your shoulders. Reposition your feet as needed to allow full extension of your body. Do not allow the ribcage or low back to sag toward the floor or the hips to hike up toward the ceiling.

Exhale. Shift your weight back toward the wall behind you. This will cause your hips to rise up in the air forming an inverted V position. Your head should be aligned with your spine or slightly tucked. Try not to lift the head. Press your heels toward the floor. If your hamstrings are tight, you may allow a slight bend in the knees. Work toward straight knees, reaching the heels toward the floor.

Inhale and return your body to the starting push-up position, maintaining the alignment of all your body segments.

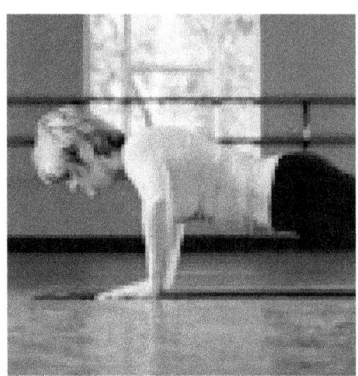

"Push up"- This classic exercise is great for your chest, arms, and shoulders. Come to a hands and knees position (quadruped) on the mat with your hands directly under your shoulders; fingers facing forward, or slightly inward and knees under your hips. Engage the abdominals and pull the shoulder blades down your back.

Reach one leg out and away followed by the other leg, bringing you to plank position. Keep the abdominals/core engaged to brace the torso. Your head should be aligned with your spine. Your feet are together with your toes tucked under and your heels reaching toward the wall behind you.

Slowly bend the elbows, lowering your body toward the floor. Keep the torso rigid and the head aligned with your spine. Do not allow your low back or ribcage to sag or your hips to hike upward. Engage your butt (glutes) and thigh (quadriceps) muscles to help maintain stability and a rigid body. Try to lower yourself until your chest or chin touch the mat or floor. Your elbows should stay close to the sides of your body or be allowed to flare outwards slightly.

Press upward through your arms, straightening the elbows. Keep the torso rigid and head aligned with your spine. Imagine pushing the floor away from you. Do not allow your low back to sag or your hips to hike upward.

An alternative position is to keep your fingers facing forward and your elbows close to your sides during the downward phase. This shifts the emphasis from the chest muscles onto the triceps and may reduce stresses in the shoulder joint.

Pushing through the outside surface and heel of your palm provides greater force in your press and stability to your shoulders.

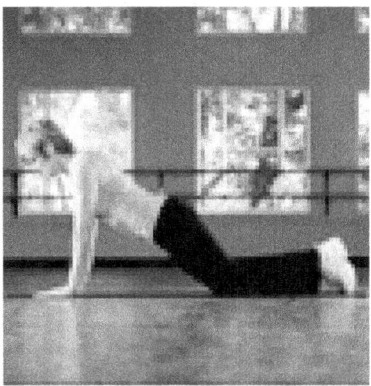

"Bent Knee Push up"- A great substitute for the push up that targets the chest, arms, and shoulders. Come to a hands and knees position on the mat with your hands directly under your shoulders; fingers facing forward and knees under your hips. Engage the abdominals and pull the shoulder blades down your back.

Reposition your knees as needed to create a straight line in your body from the knees, through the torso and out through the head. There should be no bend at the hips. Keep the abdominals braced.

Keeping the torso rigid and head aligned with your spine, slowly bend your elbows and lower your body toward the floor. Do not allow your low back to sag or your hips to hike upward. Continue to lower yourself until your chest or chin touch the mat or floor. Your elbows should remain close to the sides of your body or flare outwards slightly.

Maintaining a rigid torso and head aligned with your spine, press upward through your arms. Do not allow your low back to sag or your hips to hike upward. Continue pressing until the elbows are straight. Push-ups place stress upon the wrist joints. To alleviate some of this stress you may opt to use dumbbells and grip the handles rather than place your hands on the floor. If you are pressing from an elevation such as a dumbbell, you do not need to lower your chest or chin to the floor, but rather lower yourself until your chest or chin are level with the dumbbell handles.

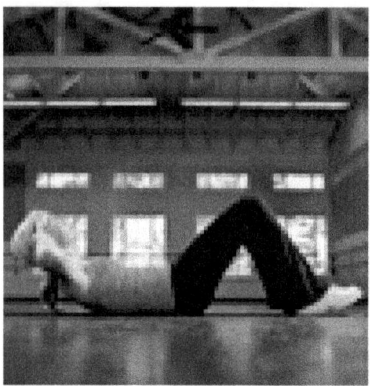

"Bent Knee Sit up"- This classic exercise focuses on your abs. Lie on your back on a mat with your knees bent, feet flat on the floor and heels a comfortable distance (12-18") away from your seat.

Place your hands behind your head. Pull your shoulder blades together and your elbows back without arching your low back or causing your ribs to splay out. This elbow position should be maintained throughout the exercise. Your head should be aligned with your spine.

Exhale. Engage your abdominal and core muscles. Nod your chin slightly as you slowly curl your head and shoulders off the mat. Pull your rib cage together and toward your pelvis. Keep the neck relaxed. Your feet, tailbone and lower back should remain in contact with the mat at all times. Continue curling up until your upper back is lifted off the mat. Hold this position briefly.

Gently inhale and lower your torso back toward the mat slowly and with control. Keep your feet, tailbone and low back in contact with the mat. Proper form is important for this exercise to prevent excessive stress on your low back. Individuals typically perform this movement too rapidly and recruit the hip flexors to assist with the upward phase. Doing this should be avoided as it causes the pelvis to tilt anteriorly, increasing the stress on the low back. The abdominals connect the rib cage to the pelvis so the movement should focus on bringing these two body parts closer together while keeping the neck and shoulders relaxed.

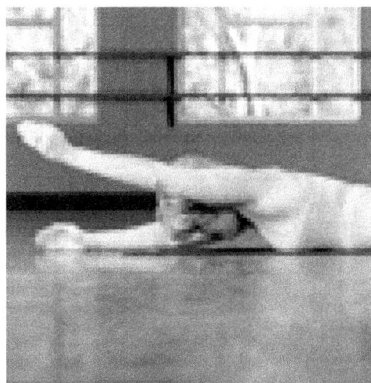

"Contralateral Limb Raises"- This simple exercise tones your back, hips, and shoulders. Lie on your stomach on a mat or the floor with your legs outstretched behind you. Your toes are pointing toward the wall behind you. Reach your arms out overhead with your palms facing each other. Keep your head aligned with your spine.

Exhale. Deepen your abdominal/core muscles to stabilize your spine and slowly float one arm a few inches off the floor. Keep your arm straight and try not to rotate your arm or shoulder. Your head and torso should not move, avoid any arching in your back. Do not lift your chin or lower your head. Hold this position briefly.

Gently inhale and lower your arm back towards your starting position without any movement in your low back or hips.

From your starting position, deepen your abdominal and core muscles to stabilize your spine and slowly stretch leg out and allow the leg to lift off of the floor. Keep your leg straight and your toes reaching to the wall behind you. Keep both hip bones and pubic bone in contact with the mat. Avoiding any rotation in your leg or pelvis. Your head and torso should not move, avoiding any arching in your back. Do not lift your chin or lower your head. Hold this position briefly. Return to your starting position.

From your starting position, deepen your abdominal/core muscles to stabilize your spine. Reach one leg out and way until it lifts off the floor. At the same time float the opposite arm a few inches off the floor. Keep both your leg and arm straight and avoid any rotation in either. Your head and torso should not move, avoiding any arching in your back. Do not lift your chin or lower your head. Hold this position briefly. Return to your starting position.

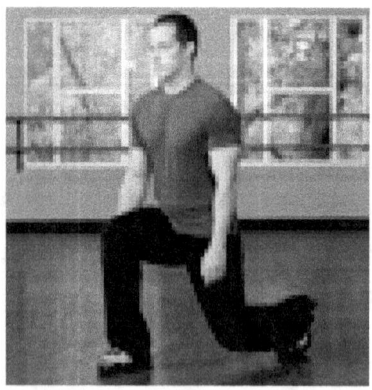

"Forward Lunge"- This good exercise helps your abs, hips, and thighs. Stand with your feet together. Pull your shoulder blades toward your hips. Engage your abdominal/core muscles ("brace") to stabilize your spine.

In preparation to step forward, slowly lift one foot off the floor and find your balance on the standing leg. Try not to move the standing foot and maintain balance without wobbling. Pause. Hold this position briefly before stepping forward. The raised foot should land on the heel first. Slowly shift your body weight onto the lead foot, placing it firmly on the floor. As you shift your body weight to the lead foot/leg, avoid the tendency to tilt or sway the upper body and try not to move the forward foot.

As you step forward into the lunge, focus on a downward movement of your hips toward the floor. Avoid driving your hips forward. This will help control the forward movement of your shinbone over your foot. Continue lowering your body to a comfortable position or until your front thigh becomes parallel with the floor and your shinbone is in a slight forward lean. During the movement, slightly bend forward at your hips. Keep the back straight.

Firmly push off with the front leg, activating both your thighs and butt muscles to return to your upright, starting position.

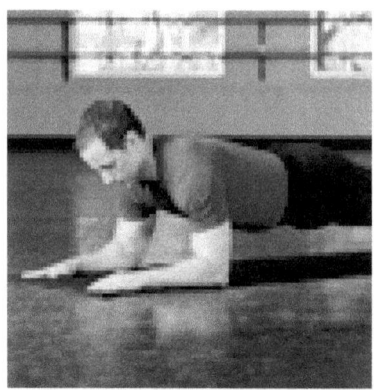

"Forward Plank"- Lie on your stomach on an exercise mat or floor with your elbows close to your sides and directly under your shoulders, palms down and fingers facing forward. Engage your abdominal/core muscles. It should feel like you are tightening a corset around your ribs, waist and lower torso. Contract your thigh muscles to straighten your legs strongly and flex your ankles, (tucking your toes towards your shins).

Slowly lift your torso and thighs off the floor or mat. Keep your torso and legs rigid. Do not allow any sagging in your ribcage or low back. Avoid hiking your hips into the air or bending the knees. Keep the shoulders away from the ears (no shrugging). The shoulders should be directly over your elbows with your palms facing down through the entire exercise. Continue to breathe, keeping the abdominals strong while holding this position. Try holding this position for 5 seconds or more.

Keep the torso and legs stiff as you slowly and gently lower your body back towards the mat or floor.

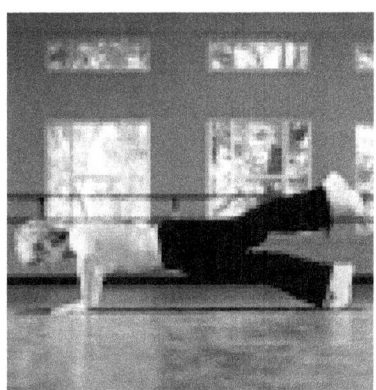

"Push-up with Single-leg Raise"- This advanced push up helps your arms, chest, shoulders, and hips. Come to a hands and knees position (quadruped) on the mat with your hands directly under your shoulders; fingers facing forward, and knees under your hips. Engage the abdominals and pull the shoulder blades down your back.

Reach one leg out and away followed by the other leg, bringing you to plank position. Keep the abdominals/core engaged to brace the torso. Your head should be aligned with your spine. Your feet are together with your toes tucked under and your heels reaching toward the wall behind you

Slowly bend the elbows, lowering your body toward the floor. Keep the torso rigid and the head aligned with your spine. Do not allow your low back or ribcage to sag or your hips to hike upward. Engage your glutes (butt) and quadriceps (thigh) muscles to help maintain stability and a rigid body. Try to lower yourself until your chest or chin touch the mat or floor. Your elbows should remain close to the sides of your body or be allowed to flare outwards slightly.

Straighten the elbows, pressing upward through your arms. Keep the torso rigid and head aligned with your spine. As you straighten the arms, lift your left foot off the floor, keeping the knee straight. Do not allow the hips to rotate as you raise the leg off the floor. Do not allow your low back or ribcage to sag or your hips to hike upward. Continue pressing until the elbows are straight and your left leg is off the floor. Hold this position briefly before returning to your starting position. Repeat the push up alternating legs with each repetition.

Pushing through the heel and outside surface of your palm provides greater force in your press and stability to your shoulders.

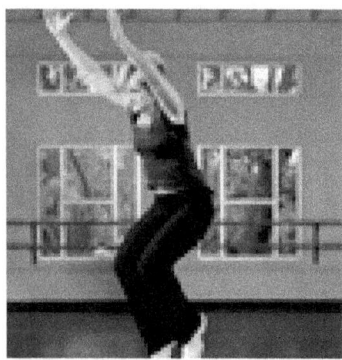

"Squat Jumps"- This bursting exercise centers on your hips and thighs. Stand with your feet hip-width apart, arms by your sides. Pull your shoulder blades down and engage your abdominal / core muscles to brace your spine.

Shift your hips back and down. This will create a hinge-like movement at your knees. Continue to lower yourself until you feel your heels about to lift off the floor. Try to maintain a flat back by bending forward at the hips. Keep your head directly facing forward and position your arms where they offer the greatest degree of balance support.

With ONLY a very brief pause at the bottom of your downward phase, explode up through your lower body, fully extending your hips, knees and ankles. As your jump into the air, try to keep your feet level with each other and parallel with the floor.

The most important components of the landing phase are correct foot position and avoiding excessive forward movement in your lower extremity, which places additional stress on your knees.

Try to land softly and quietly on the mid-foot, rolling into the heels. Always push your hips back and down to absorb the impact of landing. Do not lock out your knees on your landing.

Land with your trunk slightly forward, head aligned with your spine and back rigid or flat. Keep your abdominal / core muscles engaged, bracing your torso to protect your spine.

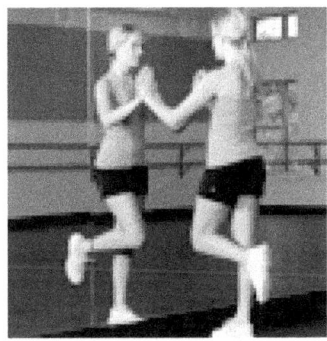

"Standing Calf Raises"- This exercise focuses on your calves and shins. Stand 6 -12" away from a wall with your feet hip-width apart and toes facing forward. Place your hands on the wall, shoulder height.

Exhale. Slowly rise up on to your toes, lifting your heels off the floor. Keep your knees straight. Do not allow the feet to rotate. Use your hands on the wall to support your balance. Hold the raised position briefly.

Inhale and slowly lower your heels back to the floor.

Exercise Variation: Single-leg Calf Raise: From your starting position, bend your left knee to lift your left foot off the floor. Perform single-leg calf raises. Repeat with your right leg.

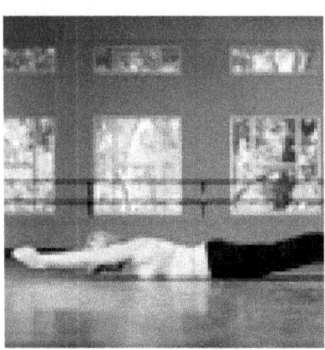

"Superman"- This "superhuman" stretch focuses on your hips, back, and arms. Lie on your stomach on a mat or the floor with your legs outstretched behind you. Your toes are pointing toward the wall behind you. Reach your arms out overhead with your palms facing each other. Relax your neck and align your head with your spine.

Exhale. Deepen your abdominal and core muscles to stabilize your spine and slowly and strongly reach both legs away from your torso until they lift a few inches off the floor. At the same time float both arms a few inches off the floor. Keep both legs and arms straight and allow any rotation in the arms, legs, shoulders or pelvis. Your head is aligned with your spine. Do not allow your head to lift up or to droop toward the floor. Do not allow the back to arch. Hold this position briefly.

Gently inhale and lower your legs and arms back to your starting position without any movement in your low back or hips.

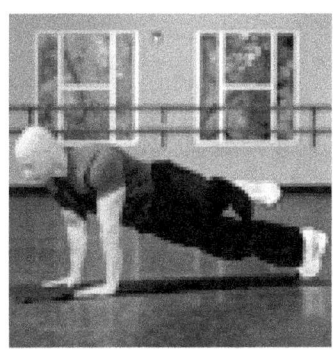

"Hip Rotations (push up position)"- This advanced exercise utilizes your abs, hips, and thighs. This exercise is a dynamic movement exercise used to prepare the body for activity. As it involves a modification to a traditional push-up, it is highly recommended you master your push-up technique before attempting this exercise.

Kneel on an exercise mat and bring your feet together behind you. Slowly bend forward to place your palms flat on the mat, positioning your hands shoulder-width apart with your fingers facing forward or turned slightly inward. Slowly shift your weight forward until your shoulders are positioned directly over your hands. Reposition your hands as needed to allow full extension of your body without any bend at the hips or knees. Brace your torso by engaging your abdominal / core muscles. Contract your glutes and quadriceps (butt and thigh muscles), and align your head with your spine. Place your feet together with your toes tucked towards your shins.

Rotational Movement: Exhale and gently draw one knee up toward its corresponding armpit. Do NOT allow your hips and low back to pitch upwards or sag down towards the floor.

In this knee-tuck position, rotate your hips to move your bent knee across the front of your torso toward its opposite armpit. Do not hike or drop your hips. Continue to move until your hips cannot rotate any further. Your head and shoulder should remain level throughout the exercise. Pause very briefly.

Rotate the hip in the opposite direction (away from your torso), until your hips cannot rotate any further without movement in your spine. Your bent knee is pointing away from your body. Your head and shoulder should remain level throughout the exercise.

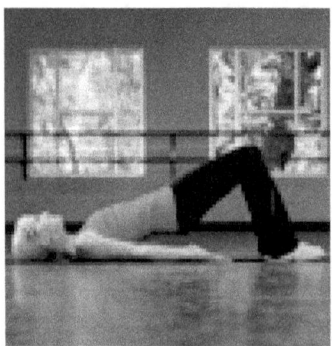

"Glute Bridge"- This bridge helps tighten your hips and abs. Lie on your back on an exercise mat or the floor in a bent-knee position with your feet flat on the floor. Place your feet hip-width apart with the toes facing away from you. Gently contract your abdominal muscles to flatten your low back into the floor. Attempt to maintain this gentle muscle contraction throughout the exercise.

Gently exhale. Keep the abdominals engaged and lift your hips up off the floor. Press your heels into the floor for added stability. Avoid pushing your hips too high, which can cause hyperextension (arching) in your low back. Keeping your abdominals strong helps to prevent excessive arching in the low back.

Inhale and slowly lower yourself back to your starting position.

Gradually progress this exercise by starting with both feet together and extending one leg while in the raised position.
Avoid arching your low back as you press your hips upward, which normally occurs if you attempt to push your hips as high as possible. This can be achieved by contracting your abdominal muscles prior to lifting, and keeping them engaged throughout the lift

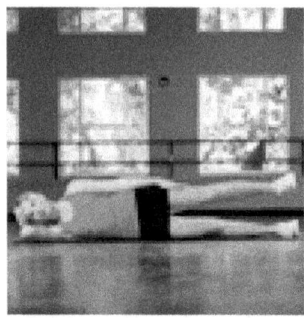

"Side Lying Hip Abduction"- This exercise focuses on your hips. Lie on your side on a mat/floor with your legs lengthened straight away from your body. Stack your feet in neutral position. Your lower arm can be bent and placed under your head for support. Your upper arm rests upon your upper hip. Your hips and shoulders should be stacked up and aligned vertically to the floor. Your head should be aligned with your spine. Engage your abdominal muscles to support your spine.

Exhale. Gently raise the upper leg off the lower leg. Keep the knee straight and the foot in a neutral position. Do not allow the hips to roll forward or back. Both knees should be "looking" straight ahead. Continue raising the leg until the hips begin to tilt, the waist collapses into the floor or until your feel tension develop in your low back or oblique muscles.

Gently inhale and return the leg to your starting position in a slow, controlled manner. After completing your set, roll over and repeat with the opposite leg.

A common mistake is raising the leg too high in this exercise. Given the design of the hip joint, the thigh can only abduct (move out sideways) to 45 degrees. Any movement beyond that position involves movement of the entire hip and no longer targets the muscles intended for this exercise.

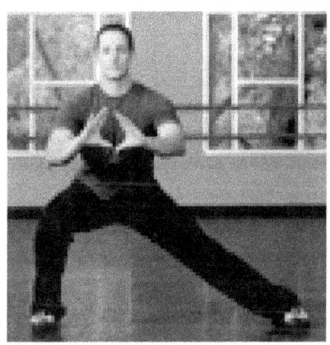

"Side Lunge"- This helps your hips and thighs. Stand with your feet parallel, hip-width apart. Your hands are in a comfortable position to help you maintain your balance during the exercise. Keep your head over your shoulder and your chin tipped and slightly upward. Shift your weight onto your heels. Engage your abdominals to stabilize the spine. Pull the shoulder blades down and back. Try to maintain these engagements throughout the exercise.

Inhale and slowly step to the right while keeping your weight into your left heel. Both feet are still facing forward. Once your right foot is firmly placed on the floor, begin to shift your weight toward the right foot, bending the right knee and pushing the hips back. Continue to lunge until your shinbone is vertical to the floor and your right knee is aligned with the second toe of your right foot. Your left leg should be as straight as possible and your body weight should be distributed into the right hip. The heels of both feet should stay flat on the floor. Your arms can be positioned where necessary to help maintain your balance.

Exhale and push off firmly with your right foot, returning to starting position. Repeat the movement for the opposite side.

Exercise variation: Reaching for your right foot with your left hand will emphasize hip flexion (alternate with the right hand reaching for the left foot).

A common mistake when performing a side lunge is that individuals often step too wide and are unable to align the shinbone over the placed foot and the knee falls inside the foot. In this case, simply take a smaller step to allow you to align the shinbone over the placed foot.

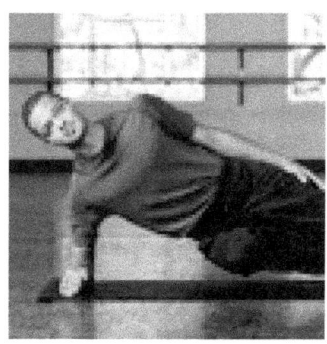

"Side Plank"- This helps your hips and thighs. Lie on your right side on an exercise mat with your legs straight and the left leg stacked directly on top of the right. Bend the right elbow and place it directly under your shoulder. Bend your right knee to about 90 degrees. The left leg stays straight with the side of your left foot resting on the mat. Align your head with your spine.

Exhale, keep the abdominals engaged to brace the spine. Your head should be aligned with your spine and your right elbow should stay directly under your shoulder. With the abdominals engaged, raise your torso off the mat, coming to support yourself on your right forearm. Your hips and right knee are in contact with the exercise mat.

Inhale and gently return yourself to your starting position. After a prescribed number of repetitions, repeat on the other side.

Exercise Variation: Increase the intensity of the exercise by increasing the length of time you are in the raised position.
Any excessive pressure on the inside of your upper foot or upper knee may cause undesirable stresses on those joints and merits termination of this exercise.

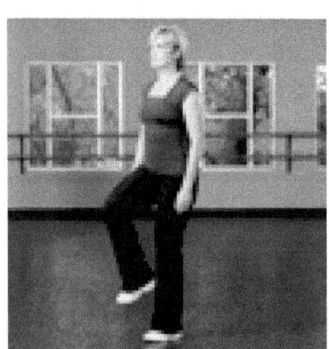

"Single Leg Stand"- This is great for abs. Stand with both feet together or spread a few inches apart (2-3"), and parallel with each other. Pull your shoulder blades down your back and engage your abdominal muscles to stabilize the spine. Bend your knees slightly and keep tension in your inner and outer thigh muscles. This will help control the tendency to shift sideways during the single-leg stand.

Slowly lift one leg 3-6" off the floor; find your balance on the standing leg. Avoid any sideways tilting or swaying in your upper body and try not to move the standing foot. Hold for 10-15 seconds before returning the foot to the floor. Perform an equal number of repetitions with each foot.

Exercise Variation: Increase the intensity of this exercise by going through the following progressions (1) lift the one leg higher off the floor (illustrated) to further raise your center of mass, (2) raise both arms overhead (3) lift one arm to your side, (4) tilt your head, (5) close your eyes then finally (6) close your eyes and tilt your head.

Try to perform this exercise in front of a mirror initially so that you can watch and control the degree sideways shift over the standing leg. Always try to minimize the shifting the hips as it places excessive stress on your knee joint. While balancing on the standing leg, think about pressing your foot into the floor and squeezing your glutes (butt muscles), this will help reduce any sideways tilting.

Most of us can lift one leg, but the question of the quality of movement is important. Perform your movements slowly and under control, avoiding any sudden positional changes. Perform each progression until you can execute them with good control and form.

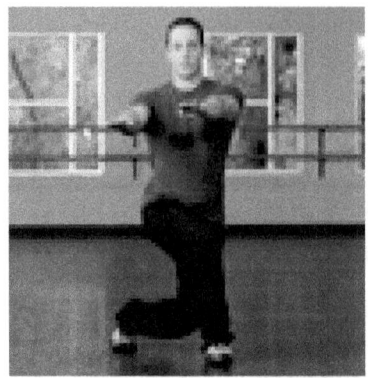

"Glute Activation Lunges"- This is killer for the abs, hips, and thighs. Stand with your feet together and your arms raised in front to shoulder height; elbows straight. Pull your shoulders down and back toward your hips. Engage your abdominal/core muscles ("brace") to stabilize your spine.

From the starting position, imagine that you are standing on a clock facing 12 o'clock. With your right foot, step across your body (both feet remain pointed forward) to the 3 o'clock position. Once the right foot is firmly placed on the floor, begin to bend at the hips. Push the hips backwards as you shift your weight over your right foot. Continue shifting your weight until your shinbone is straight up and down and your right knee is aligned directly over the second toe of your right foot. Your left knee is bent and the left heel is off the ground.

As you lunge, rotate your arms and torso in the opposite direction of the lunge movement. This increases the load on your glute muscle group. Firmly push off with your front leg, activating both your thighs and butt muscles to return to your upright, starting position.

This series of multi-directional (multi-planar) lunges are intended to activate your glutes, which protect your knee during walking, running and jumping-type activities. As many of us have weak glutes, this exercise can be performed as part of your pre-exercise warm-up. Given the moderate degree of complexity of the three movements, we recommend learning this exercise first without your arms and only progress to the arm drivers as you feel comfortable. It is suggested you first learn how to perform single leg-stands on the ground and forward lunges before performing these glute activation lunges.

These exercises should help you figure out a routine for yourself which will benefit whatever you need. For example, if you are looking to tone your abs, utilize the activities that help with abs. Don't try and do everything, it is better to have a low volume, high intensity workout than have a routine with scattered beneficence.

Chapter Four
Planning Goals/ Developing Healthy Habits

You have learned the basic essentials to creating a healthy environment for you, explored the depths of your body, heart, and mind, and have learned some exercises that you can uses for your benefit. The only thing left before you start your journey into fitness enlightenment, you must plan goals and develop healthy habits. Having a goal helps you organize and plan what you're going to do next. It's aimless to not have a goal then you have nothing to work towards which will mean that you will lose motivation, we don't want that to happen. It's even healthy to set small goals at first so they are easier to achieve until you really get the ball going and start going for the bigger goals. You must work hard and strong, you must persevere in order reach your set goal.

Ways to set a goal and keep a reminder of it are:

- You should envision how you would like to see yourself a certain amount of time from the day you started and find a way to incorporate the right amount of workouts in to help you succeed.
- You can have a calendar on your office wall primarily for your workout routine. You can fill out all the days before hand so it can tell you what you need to do the day of.
- Having sticky notes laid out everywhere to remind you to work out that day.
- Setting reminders on your cellphone will help you remember when you need to set some time aside.

Once you've found a goal and a system that works for you, you should start developing some good habits to maximize the efficiency of your plan. Good habits would mean healthier foods, lots of hydration, healthy thoughts, and so on. It is better to eat lean meals with protein and carbohydrates than eat fried meals with sugar and fat. Water is a key source to exercise. Water keeps your body hydrated which in turn keeps your body running smoothly so you can live a good life.

Maintaining a workout routine is harder than it seems, it requires a lot of dedication, For instance, you may skip one day and think that it'll be okay if you skip one more, the, you'll keep skipping days and the goal will disappear. You need to be consistent with your days and understand that it will get hard, you may want to quit, but you have to push on. One day when you've reached one of your major set goals and you're sitting in your office working, you'll look around and realize that you've got a good thing going for you. Who else can say that they've got a gym right in their office? Have fun exercising in your office!

Works Cited

Vickey, T. (n.d.). Fitness Programs | Top 25 At-Home Exercises. Retrieved August 30, 2014, from http://www.acefitness.org/acefit/fitness-programs-article/2863/Top-25-At-Home-Exercises/

http://www.spine-health.com/conditions/depression/stress-related-back-pain

http://www.mayoclinic.org/healthy-living/fitness/in-depth/exercise/art-20048389